Nursing School Success

Tools for Constructing Your Future

Donamarie Wilfong, RN, MSN
Christy Szolis, RN, MSNL
Carol Haus, RN, PhD, CNE

JONES AND BARTLETT PUBLISHERS

Sudbury, Massachusetts

BOSTON   TORONTO   LONDON   SINGAPORE

World Headquarters
Jones and Bartlett Publishers
40 Tall Pine Drive
Sudbury, MA 01776
978-443-5000
info@jbpub.com
www.jbpub.com

Jones and Bartlett Publishers Canada
6339 Ormindale Way
Mississauga, Ontario L5V 1J2
CANADA

Jones and Bartlett Publishers International
Barb House, Barb Mews
London W6 7PA
UK

Jones and Bartlett's books and products are available through most bookstores and online booksellers. To contact Jones and Bartlett Publishers directly, call 800-832-0034, fax 978-443-8000, or visit our website, www.jbpub.com.

Substantial discounts on bulk quantities of Jones and Bartlett's publications are available to corporations, professional associations, and other qualified organizations. For details and specific discount information, contact the special sales department at Jones and Bartlett via the above contact information or send an email to specialsales@jbpub.com.

Production Credits

Executive Editor: Kevin Sullivan
Acquisitions Editor: Emily Ekle
Production Director: Amy Rose
Associate Editor: Amy Sibley
Editorial Assistant: Patricia Donnelly
Production Editor: Tracey Chapman
Senior Marketing Manager: Katrina Gosek
Associate Marketing Manager: Rebecca Wasley

Manufacturing and Inventory
  Coordinator: Amy Bacus
Composition: WestWords, Inc.
Cover Design: Kristin E. Ohlin
Cover Image: © Photos.com
Printing and Binding: Malloy, Inc.
Cover Printing: Malloy, Inc.

Library of Congress Cataloging-in-Publication Data
Wilfong, Donamarie.
  Nursing school success : tools for constructing your future /
Donamarie Wilfong, Christy Szolis, Carol Haus.
    p. ; cm.
  Includes index.
  ISBN-13: 978-0-7637-4641-4 (pbk.)
  ISBN-10: 0-7637-4641-X (pbk.)
  1. Nursing—Study and teaching.　I. Szolis, Christy.　II. Haus, Carol.
III. Title.
  [DNLM: 1. Education, Nursing—Programmed Instruction.
2. Students, Nursing—Programmed Instruction. WY 18.2 W677n
2007]
  RT71.W55 2007
  610.73071—dc22

                             2006028240

6048

Printed in the United States of America
11 10 09 08 07　10 9 8 7 6 5 4 3 2 1

This book is dedicated to
My husband Donald and my sons Joshua, Jordan, and Jacob
Thank you for all your support.
I love you.
Dona

To my sons Patrick and Alec
You are my angels.
I love you.
Christy

To my sons Scott and Jeff
I love you.
Carol

And to all of our past and future students
You showed us the way.
Thank you!

Dona, Christy, and Carol

Contents

Preface

Nursing School Success: Tools for Constructing Your Future is a comprehensive, self-paced text that will help you develop the skills necessary to be a successful nursing student and a lifelong learner. Any student beginning a career in an allied health field can use this book, written for the beginning nursing student.

KEY FEATURES:

- This three-dimensional text can be used in a traditional classroom setting, as a programmed text, or as a self-paced individualized instruction workbook.
- Represented by a highlighted section of a hospital icon, each chapter introduces a new learning objective.
- Each highlighted section builds upon the other to construct a successful nursing career.
- Chapters contain learning tools for students to practice the strategies presented.
- Review questions are provided.
- Building bricks, found throughout the book, add interactive tips for successful study/learning strategies.
- Frequent breaks are included to keep you healthy.

Introduction

Constructing your future in nursing school is not always easy. There are many lessons to be learned, obstacles to overcome, and challenges to face. We, too, have built a nursing career. There are bits of information we have discovered, pieces of knowledge and strategies we have learned, that made our school years easier. We wish to share them with you and shed some light on your career-building. Our hope is that *Nursing School Success* will be your friend, your mentor, and your guide for *Constructing Your Future.*

Good luck building a nursing career.

Dona, Christy, and Carol

Chapter 1

Quality of a Nursing Student

AFTER BUILDING BRICK #1, THE STUDENT WILL BE ABLE TO:

- Identify the qualities necessary to be a successful nursing student.
- Identify the effects of staying healthy for his or her career success.

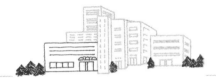

A successful nursing student:

- accepts personal responsibility.
- is a lifelong learner.
- gains self-awareness.
- takes purposeful actions.
- has a motivating factor.
- demonstrates interdependence.
- **BELIEVES IN HIM- OR HERSELF.**

A struggling nursing student:

- does not accept personal responsibility.
- views learning as boring.
- makes choices unconsciously.
- procrastinates.
- has resentments about direction in life.
- rejects assistance from others.
- **doubts his or her personal value.**

If you possess any of the features of the successful nursing student, you have the right blueprints to be a

SUCCESS!

Beginning nursing school can and should be one of the most exciting and personally enriching experiences of your life. However, it can also be one of the most stressful times. Constructing a career in nursing might not always be easy. There might be blueprint changes or unexpected delays. You will be required not only to study the theory material presented in class, but also learn many complex skills and apply this to the clinical setting. Therefore, you try to juggle all of this work into a short period. As a result, you become overwhelmed. You need to take care of yourself. As you construct your career in nursing, we will ask you to take frequent breaks. Remember:

A successful nursing student is a healthy nursing student.

As you construct your nursing career, we ask that you take the necessary breaks each day.

Stop, rest, and:

1. Exercise. Go for a walk, jog around the block, play a game of basketball, dance, or run wild!
2. Eat a healthy snack. Did you skip dinner? Maybe lunch? What about breakfast? EAT NOW!
3. Close your eyes and take a quick fantasy trip to a beautiful, peaceful place. (Take us with you.)
4. Meditate. Find a quiet, relaxing spot or thought—focus on something (not nursing).
5. Take a slow deep breath. Inhale. Exhale. Another one. One more. Feeling better?
6. Keep your chin up. Remember, no pain, no gain.
7. Have fun! Laugh! Nursing school can be fun.
8. Have positive thoughts. Say to yourself or say aloud, "I can and will do this . . ."

After laying the last brick, you will have achieved the timeless reward of

BEING A NURSE!

NOTES

NOTES

NOTES

_____
_____
_____
_____
_____
_____
_____
_____
_____
_____
_____
_____
_____
_____
_____
_____
_____
_____
_____
_____
_____
_____
_____
_____
_____
_____
_____
_____
_____
_____
_____
_____

Organization/Time Management Skills

AFTER BUILDING BRICK #2, THE STUDENT WILL BE ABLE TO:

- Recognize the importance of time management and organizational skills.
- Identify his or her time management and organizational needs.
- Learn the strategies necessary to meet time management and organizational needs.

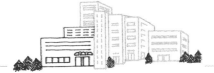

ESSENTIAL ELEMENTS

Effective time management and organizational skills provide you with a greater sense of control over your life as you meet the academic, social, and personal demands of a rigorous nursing program. Once this has been experienced, you will feel a greater satisfaction with your own accomplishments. A simple and easy-to-follow time management and organizational system is crucial to your success as a student.

IDENTIFY TIME MANAGEMENT NEEDS

- The first step in developing a time management program is to know yourself. Identify how you actually spend your time.
- Effective time management includes finding a balance between time allotted for required tasks and leisure activities.
- Complete the form "Guide for Identifying Time Management Needs" to help you achieve this balance.

SET GOALS

- Identify all the tasks you need to do for the month by completing the "Monthly Time Management Schedule."
- Effective time managers establish semester and monthly schedules.
- Allow for periodic changes in this schedule.

PRIORITIZE GOALS

- Determine the importance of each task.
- Decide how difficult the task is.
- Decide how much time each task will take.
- Determine the due date for each task.

WHY DO I NEVER GET THINGS DONE?

- No clear goals
- No priorities

- No plan
- Too many interruptions

You can get things done
beginning now . . .

DEVELOP A SCHEDULE AND MEET IT!

- Complete the Weekly Planner.
- Include a breakdown of the monthly schedule.
- Break large assignments into small steps, giving yourself adequate time to meet your deadline.
- Complete daily the Time Management Form.
- Categorize tasks into primary tasks and secondary tasks. Primary tasks are those that need to be completed that day. Secondary tasks are those that you would like to address but could be put off for a different day.
- Document estimated time to complete the task, time of day you will do the task, the time you began and completed the task, and how long it actually took you to complete it.

HOW TIME MANAGEMENT SKILLS HELP YOU GET THINGS DONE

- You get more things done in less time.
- You avoid Time Traps.
- You have more control of your life and free time too!
- You avoid time conflicts.
- You can evaluate your progress.
- You will reach your GOALS.
- You will be a better learner and a better student.

Why work harder? Just manage time to work smarter!

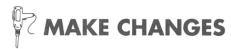

REVIEW AND EVALUATE

MAKE CHANGES

- Once all of this information is recorded, you can easily see:
  what tasks were required.
  what tasks you attempted.
  the actual time it took to complete the task.
- You can then make changes in your monthly, weekly, and daily schedule if you have not completed your tasks.

GUIDE FOR IDENTIFYING TIME MANAGEMENT NEEDS

Place a check in the box next to each item if you exhibit this behavior on a regular and consistent basis. Summarize the areas of need to complete the guide.

- ❑ You cannot complete assignments at school on time.
- ❑ Assignments are unorganized and sloppy in their appearance.
- ❑ You are unable to develop time schedules.
- ❑ You do not keep your time schedules.
- ❑ You do not understand how important time management is to being successful.
- ❑ You have difficulty reorganizing tasks.
- ❑ You do not meet the scheduled time lines for meeting personal goals.
- ❑ You do not accept the responsibility for your own time management.
- ❑ You do not learn from errors made in past time management issues.
- ❑ You take too much time to complete simple tasks.

GETTING STARTED WITH TIME MANAGEMENT

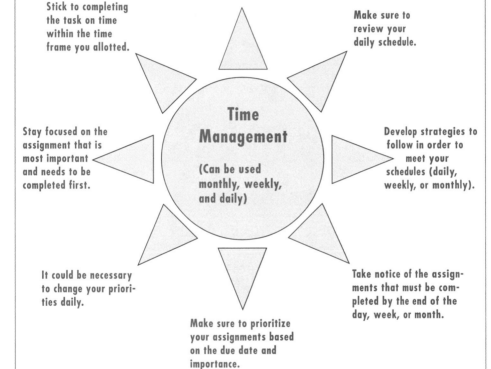

Formulate a chart for keeping track of the activities completed . . . (daily, weekly, and monthly).

Stick to completing the task on time within the time frame you allotted.

Make sure to review your daily schedule.

Time Management

(Can be used monthly, weekly, and daily)

Stay focused on the assignment that is most important and needs to be completed first.

Develop strategies to follow in order to meet your schedules (daily, weekly, or monthly).

It could be necessary to change your priorities daily.

Take notice of the assignments that must be completed by the end of the day, week, or month.

Make sure to prioritize your assignments based on the due date and importance.

STOP

EXERCISE
before moving on.

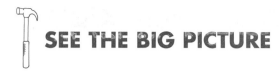

SEE THE BIG PICTURE

YOUR MONTHLY SCHEDULE FOR TIME MANAGEMENT

Fill in due dates for all assignments, papers, dates of tests, and nonacademic activities.

SUN	MON	TUE	WED	THU	FRI	SAT

WEEKLY PLANNER

MON	TUE	WED	THU	FRI	SAT/SUN

To use this planner, write times in the squares you plan to study, and how long you plan to study. Having a blank time sheet allows you to write in the times that are best for you. The schedule allows for a 7-hour day. You can adjust it to fit your needs once you get started. Also, write the topic that you will be studying at that time. Saturday and Sunday are combined if you would prefer to do half of your tasks on the different days.

DAILY TIME MANAGEMENT WORKSHEET

Primary Task	Projected Start Time	Projected Finish Time	Actual Time Taken to Complete Task

Secondary Task	Projected Start Time	Projected Finish Time	Actual Time Taken to Complete Task

DAILY PLANNING SCHEDULE

Date:_____

5:00–6:00 am_____   2:00–3:00 pm_____

6:00–7:00 am_____   3:00–4:00 pm_____

7:00–8:00 am_____   4:00–5:00 pm_____

8:00–9:00 am_____   5:00–6:00 pm_____

9:00–10:00 am_____   6:00–7:00 pm_____

10:00–11:00 am_____   7:00–8:00 pm_____

11:00–12:00 am_____   8:00–9:00 pm_____

12:00–1:00 pm_____   9:00–10:00 pm_____

1:00–2:00 pm_____   10:00–11:00 pm_____

Building Bricks

I have completed Task #1. Now what?

You have completed your first task on the list with time to spare. You contemplate whether you should start the next task. The answer to this is no. Use this time to do some things at home. Rushing into the next task can actually harm your productiveness on the next task. Instead, make use of this time to do one or more of the following:

Make a grocery list
Look at your mail
Read a book, magazine or flyer
Clean up your work area
Reorganize your daily schedule
Call some friends
Play with your children
Stretch
Have a healthy snack
Take some slow, deep breaths and relax

NOTES

NOTES

NOTES

Learning Styles/ Learning Profile

AFTER BUILDING BRICK #3, THE STUDENT WILL BE ABLE TO:

- Identify his or her learning style.
- Use the strategies necessary to meet his or her specific learning needs.

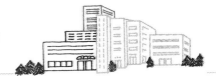

WHAT IS YOUR LEARNING STYLE?

Circle the letter that completes the following statements:

1. I remember things best when I study
   a. in the early morning.
   b. at school.
   c. in the afternoon.
   d. after dinner.
   e. late at night.

2. I study best when I am
   a. alone.
   b. with a group.
   c. with one person.
   d. sometimes alone and sometimes with a friend.
   e. with a person older than I.
   f. with the teacher.

3. I learn things best by (select all that apply)
   a. writing them down.
   b. hearing them.
   c. reading them.
   d. visualizing them.
   e. speaking them.
   f. manipulating them.

4. I learn best through
   a. my ears.
   b. my eyes.
   c. touching.
   d. a combination of _____.

5. I study best when the lighting is
   a. strong.
   b. average intensity.
   c. low.
   d. direct sunlight.

6. I concentrate best when my study area is
   a. hot.
   b. cool.
   c. warm.
   d. very cold.

7. I study best
   a. sitting at a desk.
   b. sitting in a comfortable chair.
   c. lying on the floor.
   d. lying on the bed.

8. I concentrate best when
   a. there is no noise.
   b. there is light noise in the background.
   c. the television is on.
   d. there is considerable noise.

9. I study best when I am
   a. eating as I study.
   b. hungry.
   c. chewing gum.
   d. drinking water or soda.
   e. having no food or beverages.
   f. finished eating.

10. I study best when I
    a. study for long periods of time.
    b. study for an hour.
    c. study for 30 minutes.
    d. study for 15 minutes.

LEARNING PROFILE

Look back over the answers that you circled. Now use these answers to create your own learning profile. This profile will give you a picture of how you learn best. After you have determined your learning style, turn the page to learn the strategies you need to help you be successful!

ENVIRONMENTAL NEEDS

(See Questions 5, 6, 7, 8 in the previous section)
I study best when:

the lighting is _____

the temperature is _____

the sound level is _____

the place I am working at is _____

SOCIAL NEEDS

(See Question 2 in the previous section)
I study best when I am _____

SENSORY NEEDS

(See Questions 3, 4 in the previous section)
I study best when I use the _____ sense(s), and I learn things best by _____

I study best when: _____

my study time is _____

the amount of time I study is _____

the food or drink I consume is _____

> ### Building Bricks
>
> ## Where should I study?
>
> You do not need a fancy study area, but you do need to establish one place for doing most of your studying. This place does not have to be a soundproof cell. However, it should not be a recreational area either. It does not matter if you select a study place for yourself at home, at school, or in a library as long as you usually study in the same place. It is important that you study in the same place so you do not waste time and energy adjusting to a new area or location.

Tips for Learning Best by Reading

In your reading-based classes:

- You should excel; this is your best way of learning. Make sure you keep up with the reading.

In your listening-based classes:

- Try to take careful notes, or borrow a friend's notes, and read them over frequently.
- Write out answers to questions, and then read them to learn them.
- Ask the instructor to write key concepts or words on the board.

In your speaking-based classes:

- Keep a pad of paper next to you, and write notes on what you are going to say. Then read your notes before you speak.

In your visual-based classes:

- Take notes on videos and demonstrations that you can read through later.

In your writing-based classes:

- Reread what you have written to ensure that it makes sense.

In your manipulating-based classes:

- Keep a journal of your experiences and read it to help you remember how the activities went.

In general:

- Make and use flash cards to help you learn information.
- Ask instructors to recommend articles or journals that will explain materials covered in class.

Tips for Learning Best by Writing

In your reading-based classes:

- Before you read, write down what you already know about the topic.
- Write summaries of each chapter or section after you have read it.

In your listening-based classes:

- Make sure to take careful notes, rewrite your notes, and fill in any missing pieces of information.

In your speaking-based classes:

- Write down what you want to say before you say it.

In your visual-based classes:

- Copy any visual aids or key information written on the board.
- Take notes on videos and rewrite them for review.

In your writing-based classes:

- You should excel in these classes, because this is your favorite way to learn. Make sure you hand in all your assignments on time.

In your manipulating-based classes:

- Write down the steps of the process after you have done it.
- Keep a journal of your experiences, so you can remember them later.

In general:

- Keep a small notebook with you at all times, and write down what you need to remember.

Tips for Learning Best by Listening

In your reading-based classes:

- Read anything you do not understand into a tape recorder and play it back to assist in your studying.

In your listening-based classes:

- This is your favorite way to learn. You should excel in these classes. Make sure you attend all your classes.

In your speaking-based classes:

- Make sure you listen carefully to what other students say. You can learn a lot from them.

In your visual-based classes:

- Narrate what you see into a tape recorder during or after class. Then play the tape back to assist in your studying.

In your writing-based classes:

- Read your papers aloud to yourself and make sure they sound correct.

In your manipulating-based classes:

- Listen carefully to directions and explanations. Talk yourself through activities.

In general:

- Discuss ideas aloud with yourself.
- Have someone read tests to you or read them aloud yourself.

Eat Something Healthy!

Tips for Learning Best by Speaking

In your reading-based classes:

- Read aloud and talk about the ideas as you read to yourself.

In your listening-based classes:

- Repeat major ideas from the lecture to yourself or a friend.

In your speaking-based classes:

- This is your preferred way of learning. You should excel in these classes. Make sure you attend every class.

In your visual-based classes:

- Give the "play by play" of what you see to a friend or to yourself.

In your writing-based classes:

- Speak your ideas into a tape recorder, and then transcribe what you have recorded.

In your manipulating-based classes:

- Narrate your activities. Talk about what you are doing with your project partners.
- Ask questions in class.

In general:

- Go to your instructor's office and discuss questions with him or her.
- Study by asking questions aloud and then answer them for yourself.

Tips for Learning Best by Visualizing

In your reading-based classes:

- Before you read a chapter, look at all the charts and pictures.
- As you are reading, try to picture what is happening as if it were a movie.

In your listening-based classes:

- Draw representations of what the professor is talking about, instead of just taking notes in written form.

In your speaking-based classes:

- Picture what you want to say, and then talk about what you have pictured.

In your visual-based classes:

- You should excel in these classes, because this is your preferred way of learning.

In your writing-based classes:

- Draw a representation of what you want to write about. Also, draw pictures and make diagrams to enhance your professor's understanding of your writing.

In your manipulating-based classes:

- Visualize yourself doing a task before you do it.

In general:

- Close your eyes and practice "seeing" what you need to remember.
- Make "maps" of information to help you remember it.

Tips for Learning Best by Manipulating

In your reading-based classes:

- Try out any activities described in your reading.
- Try to minimize rhythmic activities or fidgeting because they could slow down reading.

In your listening-based classes:

- Practice any concepts learned in class.
- Listen closely and then role-play the information discussed.

In your speaking-based classes:

- Participate actively in discussions.
- Demonstrate what you are talking about by manipulating objects.

In your visual-based classes:

- Pay close attention to visuals and try to re-create them or representations of them.

In your writing-based classes:

- Act out what you want to write about, and have a friend take notes on your acting.
- Use this as an outline for your writing.

In your manipulating-based classes:

- You should excel in these classes because this is your preferred way of learning.
- Volunteer to demonstrate in front of the class whenever possible.

In general:

- Make models of hard to understand concepts.
- Watch someone do something before trying it yourself.

TRAITS WORKSHEET

What Are Your Strengths?

+ - **Strength**
÷ - **Need improvement**

__Academic	__Affectionate	__Assertive	__Capable
__Accurate	__Aggressive	__Bold	__Careful
__Active	__Alert	__Broadminded	__Cautious
__Adaptable	__Ambitious	__Businesslike	__Charming
__Adventurous	__Artistic	__Calm	__Cheerful

__Clear-Thinking	__Forceful	__Modest	__Retiring
__Clever	__Formal	__Natural	__Robust
__Competent	__Frank	__Obliging	__Self-Confident
__Competitive	__Friendly	__Open-Minded	__Self-Controlled
__Confident	__Generous	__Opportunistic	__Sensible
__Conscientious	__Gentle	__Optimistic	__Sensitive
__Conservative	__Good-Natured	__Organized	__Serious
__Considerate	__Healthy	__Outgoing	__Sharp-Witted
__Cool	__Helpful	__Painstaking	__Sincere
__Cooperative	__Honest	__Patient	__Sociable
__Courageous	__Humorous	__Peaceable	__Spontaneous
__Creative	__Idealistic	__Persevering	__Spunky
__Curious	__Independent	__Pleasant	__Stable
__Daring	__Individualistic	__Poised	__Steady
__Deliberate	__Industrious	__Polite	__Strong
__Democratic	__Informal	__Practical	__Strong-Minded
__Dependable	__Ingenious	__Precise	__Sympathetic
__Dignified	__Intellectual	__Progressive	__Tactful
__Discreet	__Intelligent	__Prudent	__Teachable
__Dominant	__Inventive	__Purposeful	__Tenacious
__Eager	__Kind	__Quick	__Thorough
__Easygoing	__Leisurely	__Quiet	__Verbal
__Efficient	__Lighthearted	__Rational	__Versatile
__Emotional	__Likeable	__Realistic	__Warm
__Energetic	__Logical	__Reasonable	__Wholesome
__Enterprising	__Loyal	__Reflective	__Wise
__Enthusiastic	__Mature	__Relaxed	__Witty
__Fair-Minded	__Methodical	__Reliable	__Zany
__Farsighted	__Meticulous	__Reserved	
__Firm	__Mild	__Resourceful	
__Flexible	__Moderate	__Responsible	

On the lines below write any additional words that describe you or that other people use to describe you:

_____

_____

_____

_____

_____

_____

Using the information you learned about yourself from completing the Traits Worksheet, identify your strengths and areas of needed improvement. Now:

Set Your Goals

List four strengths you possess that will lead to your success as a nursing student.

1.
2.
3.
4.

List four areas that need improvement to help you succeed as a nursing student.

1.
2.
3.
4.

Now set three goals that are important to you for this course. These goals should be measurable. Be very specific with your goals.

1.

2.

3.

Answer the following questions honestly:

1. What makes these goals important to you? Why?

2. What do you need to change in your habits to successfully attain your goals?

NOTES

NOTES

Study Skills

AFTER BUILDING BRICK #4, THE STUDENT WILL BE ABLE TO:

- Describe the study strategies needed for success.
- Utilize specific study strategies as a learning tool.

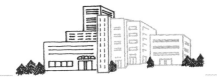

Learning how to STUDY is learning how to LEARN. This process should not be painful or boring. Strong study skills help you avoid the anxieties and pressures that go along with the many academic and clinical skills you must learn. This brick provides you with the necessary skills to be a successful lifelong learner.

WHERE DO YOU LIKE TO STUDY?

Directions:

Place a check next to the answer that best describes you. Once you have done this you will identify what type of areas work best for you. Avoid situations that do not work well for you.

    1. I learn best:
      ❏ visually.
      ❏ orally.

2. During class, I need to:
   ❑ pay close attention to taking notes.
   ❑ pay close attention to listening.
   ❑ sit in the front.
   ❑ sit near a window.
   ❑ sit near a door.
   ❑ sit in the back.

3. I study best:
   ❑ at home.
   ❑ in the library.
   ❑ somewhere else.

4. I study best:
   ❑ on weekends.
   ❑ daily.
   ❑ in the morning.
   ❑ in the afternoon.
   ❑ in the evening.

5. I study best:
   ❑ before dinner.
   ❑ after dinner.

6. I study best:
   ❑ in a group.
   ❑ alone.
   ❑ with a friend.

7. I study best:
   ❑ when I do it before I have to.
   ❑ when under pressure.
   ❑ with music.
   ❑ in a quiet area.
   ❑ when watching TV.
   ❑ in an organized study session.
   ❑ completing one subject at a time.

8. I take breaks:
   ❑ every 30 minutes.
   ❑ every hour.
   ❑ every 2 hours.
   ❑ every __ hours.

STUDY SKILLS EVALUATION

Place a check mark in the column that best describes the way you study.

STUDY PLACE	ALWAYS	SOMETIMES	NEVER	
I				study in the same place at home.
I				study in the same place at school.
I				organize my study area.
I				have supplies in my study area.
STUDY TIME	ALWAYS	SOMETIMES	NEVER	
I				follow a study schedule.
I				study every day.
I				study for more than one hour every day.
I				do my hardest assignments first.
I				review after every class.
I				review on days when I have no homework.
I				schedule a weekly review session.
BASIC STUDY SKILLS	ALWAYS	SOMETIMES	NEVER	
I				use different study methods for different subjects.

continued

	ALWAYS	SOMETIMES	NEVER	
I				concentrate when I study.
I				have a list of my daily assignments.
I				write my future assignments on a calendar.
I				use a dictionary when I study.
I				take notes when I study.
I				get help when I have trouble understanding something.
I				use the correct form when writing an outline.
CLASSROOM STUDY SKILLS	**ALWAYS**	**SOMETIMES**	**NEVER**	
I				take notes during class time.
I				review my class notes.
I				listen attentively during class discussions.
I				participate actively in class discussions.
I				use textbook aids.
I				turn in my assignments on time.

Now look back over the check marks in the different areas. If most of your answers are "always" or "sometimes," you have good study skills. For every "never" marked, keep it in mind as an area you need to improve so you will be able to apply the information to your study skills.

Building Bricks

Study Overload

When you study hard, you can "overload" and not process information.

Common signs are:

- Feeling hungry
- Yawning
- Reading the same sentence over and over
- Being unable to understand what you read
- Being easily distracted by small sounds
- Being unable to remember what you study

If you experience any of the above signs, what should you do?

- Take a short break
- Change study topics

 ## MAKING NEW STRATEGIES

Choose three study strategies and write how these strategies will work for you. Then devise a plan to use these strategies in a new way.

STRATEGY 1 PLAN

I will use this strategy by:

I will try to use this strategy in the following way:

STRATEGY 2 PLAN

I will use this strategy by:

I will try to use this strategy in the following way:

STRATEGY 3 PLAN

I will use this strategy by:

I will use this strategy in the following way:

STUDY STRATEGIES

Try these tools to help you study more efficiently.

STRATEGY	TASK AREA	PROCESS	DESCRIPTION
PIRATES	Test Taking	**P**repare to succeed. **I**nspect instructions carefully. **R**ead entire question, remember memory strategies, and reduce choices. **A**nswer question or leave until later. **T**urn back to the abandoned items. **E**stimate unknown answers by avoiding absolutes and eliminating similar choices. **S**urvey to ensure that all items have a response.	PIRATES can help learners to complete tests more carefully and successfully.
PQ4R	Reading	**P**review **Q**uestion **R**ead **R**eflect **R**ecite **R**eview	PQ4R can help students become more discriminating readers.
SCORER	Test taking	**S**chedule time effectively. **C**lue words identified. **O**mit difficult items until end. **R**ead carefully the question. **E**stimate answers requiring calculations. **R**eview work and responses.	This test-taking strategy provides a structure for completing various tests by helping students carefully and systematically complete test items.

continued

STRATEGY	TASK AREA	PROCESS	DESCRIPTION
SQRQCQ	Math word problems	Survey word problem. Question asked is identified. Read more carefully. Question process required to solve problem. Compute the answer. Question yourself to ensure that the answer solves the problem.	This strategy provides a systematic structure for identifying the question being asked in a math word problem, computing the response, and ensuring that the question in the problem was answered.
SQ3R	Reading	Survey Question Read Recite Review	SQ3R provides a systematic approach to improve reading comprehension.

When is a good time to study?

Finding a good time to study is a difficult task. Set aside some time each day to study. It is a good idea to have a set time each day and stick to that time. Some helpful hints to figure out your best study time are:

1. What are your sleeping habits? Do not exceed your limits. When your body tells you it is tired, listen to it. Studying past your limits will not increase your learning, it will actually decrease your retention of information.

2. Find out when you do your best work. In the morning, afternoon, or evening.

3. Use your downtime (less energetic time) to do less challenging tasks.

4. Change your schedule to study when you can.

STUDY GROUPS

Study groups are an underused study technique that are quite helpful. They provide the use of several modalities: reviewing information, reading, writing, and listening to others in the group.

Tips for forming a study group:

1. Include 3 to 5 students.
2. Seek diversity of experience and a common dedication.
3. Find a balance of strengths and weaknesses.
4. Begin to meet as soon as the test is announced.
5. Make meeting times and dates formal and rigorous.
6. Appoint a chairperson (rotate with each test).
7. Assign each member topics or sections according to course outline.
8. Each member prepares a summary of the topics with five questions he or she answers.
9. Answer and discuss questions.

 # THE WORKING NOTEBOOK

The Working Notebook is one of the most important organizational tools a student can have. It contains all the necessary materials to help you be a successful student. Bring it to class every day. It includes a daily schedule, course outlines, weekly learning activities, a personal calendar, handouts, and assignments. We suggest one for theory and one for clinical. Update it at the end of each course. Materials from the notebook should be dated, labeled, and stored in an accordion-type folder so you can refer to them as needed.

NOTEBOOK CHECKLIST

The following items are good to keep in a zippered pouch in your notebook:

Three-hole punch

Pens and pencils

Sticky notes

Correction fluid

Paper clips

Highlighters

Calculator

ORGANIZING YOUR WORKING NOTEBOOK:

Keep yourself organized from the beginning. Be sure to use subject dividers in your notebook to separate handouts and notes. Be sure to date your papers when you get them and file them under the correct sections of your notebook. Also carry a monthly calendar with dates. If you wait too long, you will have too much information, and you will never be organized. Organization is a great way to keep you in step with the busy life of school.

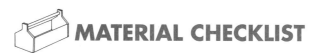 MATERIAL CHECKLIST

GENERAL MATERIALS

❑ Bookbag/backpack

❑ Pencil/pen

❑ Paper

❑ Assignment calendar

❑ Notebook

The following is a list of items that you should keep in your notebook or backpack:

Clear tape   _____
Colored paper   _____
Colored pencils   _____
Colored pens   _____
Erasers   _____
Felt-tip pens   _____
Folders   _____
Glue   _____
Highlighter pens   _____
Index cards   _____
Notebook paper   _____
Paper clips   _____
Paper punch   _____
Pencil sharpener   _____
Pencils   _____
Rubber bands   _____
Ruler   _____
Scissors   _____
Scrap paper   _____
Stapler   _____

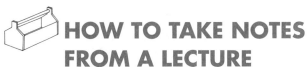

HOW TO TAKE NOTES FROM A LECTURE

1. Be prepared for each day's lecture.
   - Do all required readings prior to the lecture.
   - Review your notes from the previous lecture.
   - Utilize handouts that the instructor gives you before and during class.

2. Take organized notes and utilize the two-column form of note taking.
   - Listen attentively for the main idea of the lecture.
   - Listen for details that support the main idea.
   - Utilize shorthand and abbreviate notes so you can keep up with the lecture.
   - Use highlighters, different colored pens, and symbols to organize notes and emphasize important ideas.

TAKING TWO-COLUMN NOTES

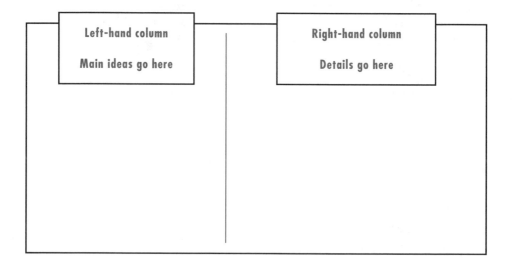

When taking notes, list all the details in the right-hand column.

- Use abbreviations. (Utilize the Shorthand Symbols Sheet.)
- Do not use a lot of words.
- Utilize markers and colored pens to draw lines connecting main ideas with details.
- Mark and underline important notes.
- Leave extra spaces between notes to add things later.
- Revise your notes within 24 hours of the lecture.
- Read over your notes and write study questions.

3. Watch your instructor.
   - Listen closely for cues that an idea might be important.
   - Take note of repeated remarks pointed out by your instructor.
   - Pay attention to your instructor's body language.
4. Pay attention and be an active listener.
   - If you cannot see or hear well, sit close to the instructor.
   - Make sure to leave space in your notes for questions that you might need to have clarified or information that you might have missed during the lecture.

STANDARD SHORTHAND SYMBOLS

Note taking can be much easier if you use the following signs and symbols for certain commonly repeated words.

$\approx$	approximately
$\rightarrow$	resulting in
$\leftarrow$	as a result of/consequence of
$+$	and or also
$>$	more than
$<$	less than
$\uparrow$	increasing
$\downarrow$	decreasing
$\subset$	it follows that
$\therefore$	therefore
$*$	most importantly
$=$	the same as
esp	especially
ff	following
cf	compare; in comparison; in relation to
w/	with

w/o	without
wh/	which
∵	because
Δ	change

THREE-STEP PROCESS FOR REVIEWING NOTES

Record

Edit

Repeat

Do these three steps within the first 24 hours of the lecture.

Record

This is the actual process of writing notes. Make sure to include the lecture notes as well as notes from the textbook.

Edit

- Check that all main ideas are recorded in the left-hand column, expressed completely and concisely.
- Check that all details are recorded on the right-hand side.
- While editing, highlight correlating information or key words; draw connecting lines and arrows; and number sequential information.

Repeat/Repeat/Repeat

1. Review both columns. (Recite verbally if needed.)
2. Cover the left column of notes and try to remember the main idea.
3. Cover the right column and try to remember details.
4. Try to correlate common factors.
5. Turn main ideas from the left column into questions with the right column being the answer.

Goal

The main goal is **AUTOMATIZATION.**

1. Learning something so thoroughly that it can be applied consistently with little or no effort.

2. When information is learned at an automatic level, you then can rely on remembering it, retrieving it from memory, and using it as a foundation for further learning.

3. Automatization includes repetition, thinking about the information, and making associations.

4. It requires constant practice and review.

Building Bricks

How to Study If You Have Children

Many students are attending school and raising families. If you have small children running around the house and you cannot concentrate on your studies, try the following tips:

1. Include the children in developing your study time schedule.

2. Have the children watch a movie or television show while you study.

3. Find someone to help watch children.

4. Plan activities for children to do to keep them busy.

NOTES

NOTES

NOTES

5

Graphic Organizers

- Define the concepts of graphic organizers.
- Describe and utilize the different types of graphic organizers.

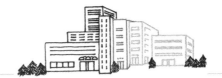

GRAPHIC ORGANIZERS

A graphic organizer is a visual representation of how ideas are related to each other. These graphic organizers help you collect information, interpret this information, problem solve, devise plans of action, and utilize critical thinking skills. Graphic organizers help you to:

1. understand how pieces of information are related.
2. increase your comprehension and recall.
3. organize your observations, research, opinions, and reflections.
4. prepare your written assignments and presentations.
5. problem solve and integrate thinking, reading, and writing processes.
6. practice critical thinking skills and apply these skills to real-world situations.

Some forms of graphic organizers are the Mind Map, Circle Chart, and the Unit Organizer. Each chart is different in appearance but similar in information gathering. There is not one preferred chart. Choose one that works best for you and meets your learning style. The following pages show examples of these types of organizers.

THE MIND MAP

The Mind Map is a study technique that uses pictures/charts/graphs to enhance memory. It increases your thinking skills by generating ideas, and composing and connecting those ideas that appear related to make a coherent whole.

Steps to creating a Mind Map:

1. List the topic in the center circle of the map.
2. Think of all the concepts that describe the topic.
3. Record the concepts in smaller circles surrounding the center circle.

MIND MAP

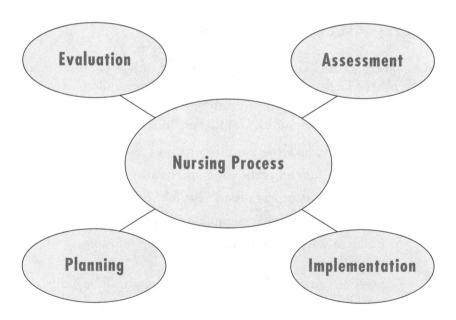

CIRCLE CHART

The Circle Chart makes distinctions among similar facts, concepts, and disease processes. It increases your thinking skills in analyzing, comparing, and contrasting.

Steps to create a Circle Chart:

1. List the topic in the center circle on the Circle Chart.
2. Write items to be compared on the lines in the individual sections.
3. Fill in facts for each item in each section.

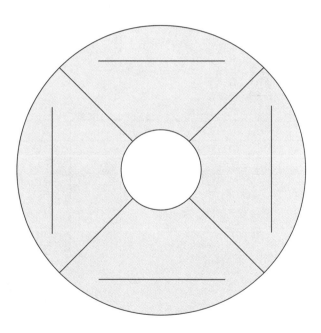

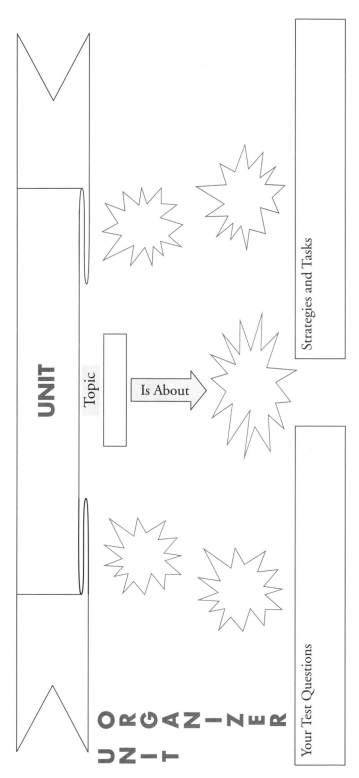

The Unit Organizer allows you to categorize according to units.
Steps to create a Unit Organizer:
1. Break down each topic in that unit.
2. Describe the content material related to each topic.
3. Formulate test questions for each topic.
4. List the strategies and tasks needed to successfully learn the material.

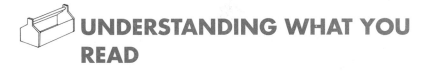

UNDERSTANDING WHAT YOU READ

1. Review during your readings to see if you understand the material or content.
2. If you do not understand what you have read, go back and reread the information.
3. Add the new information to the old information. This will broaden your knowledge base.
4. Summarize the information into your own words.

Find a Quiet Spot and Focus.

NOTES

NOTES

NOTES

Medical
Terminology

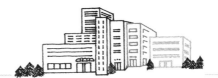

MEDICAL TERMINOLOGY

Prefix

Root

Suffix

Medical terminology is the language of the health professions. Learning this language is just as important as learning a language if you are traveling to a foreign country. You need to know it to be able to function. There are a few simple rules to learn in order to understand medical terms, as would be the case if you were studying any foreign language.

If you were fortunate enough to study Latin or Greek, you would have it made! Most medical terms derive from the Latin or Greek languages. Memorizing some common prefixes/suffixes can help you get started. You cannot learn the language overnight or even in a month. It takes exposure to new words as you read patient charts and records for you to become an expert in mastering terminology.

BASIC RULES FOR BUILDING AND DEFINING MEDICAL TERMS

The key to understanding medical terms is learning how to break the word down into smaller parts. For example, the term "erythrocyte" can be broken down into **erythro**, which means red, and **cyte,** meaning cell. Putting the two parts together, the term "erythrocyte" means red blood cell. Many times, you do not have to memorize big medical terms. If you learn to break a term down into smaller components, you can figure out what the word means.

Primarily, there are three key elements that can exist in a medical term.

- The main component of a medical term is called the **root**. It often refers to a part of the body. Some examples are:

ROOT	MEANING
cardi	heart
hepat	liver
oste	bone
my	muscle
neph	kidney

- Another component of a medical term is a **prefix**. A prefix comes in the beginning of a medical term and usually indicates a quality such as a position, number, time, amount, etc.

PREFIX	MEANING
anti	against
dys	abnormal
hyper	high, elevated
endo	inside, inner
micro	small

- A third component of a medical term is a **suffix**. A suffix comes after a root word. A suffix often indicates a disease, condition, or procedure.

SUFFIX	MEANING
algia	pain
emia	in the blood
itis	inflammation
scopy	visual exam
ectomy	removal, excision

If you read your patient's medical record and discover that he or she has **endocarditis,** you could easily figure out what this means if you have become familiar with the meanings of common prefixes, suffixes, and root words. Using the preceding lists, you could reason that **endocarditis** is an inflammation inside the heart.

endo = inside

card (i) = heart

itis = inflammation

Most medical terminology textbooks have a list of commonly used prefixes, suffixes, and roots that you can put on flash cards and memorize to get you started. Listed below is a table of common prefixes–suffixes–roots and their meanings.

PREFIX–SUFFIX–ROOT	MEANING
a(n)-	absence of
acou, acu-	hear
aden(o)-	gland
alg-	pain
angi(o)	vessel
ante-	before
anti-	against
arteri(o)-	artery
arthro-	joint
audi(o)-	hearing

continued

PREFIX–SUFFIX–ROOT	MEANING
aur(i)-	ear
bi-	two, twice
brady-	slow
carcin(o)-	cancer
cardi	heart
-centesis	puncture
cephal(o)-	head
cerebr(o)-	brain
chol(e)-	gall bladder
chondr(o)-	cartilage
circum-	around
contra-	against
cost(o)-	rib
crani(o)-	skull
cyan(o)-	blue
cyst(o)-	bladder
cyt(o)-	cell
dent-	tooth
derm	skin
dys-	abnormal, bad, difficulty
-ectomy	incision, removal
-emia	blood
encephal(o)-	brain
end(o)-	inside
enter(o)	intestine
epi-	upon, above
erythr(o)-	red
-esthesia	feeling, sensation
eu-	normal
gastr(o)	stomach
gloss(o)	tongue
glyc(o)	sweet, sugar
-gram	record
-graph	process of recording

continued

PREFIX–SUFFIX–ROOT	MEANING
gyne	woman
hemat(o)	blood
hemi-	half
hepat	liver
hist(o)	tissue
hydr(o)	water
hyper-	high, excessive
hypo-	low, deficient, under, below
hyster(o)	uterus
intra-	inside
-itis	inflammation
lapar(o)-	abdomen
leuk(o)-	white
lip(o)-	fat
-lys(is)	dissolve, destroy, loosen
mal-	bad, abnormal, poor
my	muscle
myel(o)	spinal cord, bone marrow
neph	kidney
olig(o)-	scanty
onc(o)-	tumor
oophor(o)	ovary
ophthalm(o)	eye
-opia	vision
orchi(o)	testes
-osis	condition
osse(o), oste(o)	bone
-ostomy	opening
ot(o)	ear
path(o)-	disease
ped(o)	child
-penia	deficiency
peps, pept	digest
peri-	around

continued

PREFIX–SUFFIX–ROOT	MEANING
phag(o)	eat, destroy
pharyng(o)	throat
phleb(o)	vein
-plasia	growth, formation
-phobia	fear
-plasty	repair
-plegia	paralysis
-pnea	breathing
pneum(o)	air, lung
pod(o)	foot
poly-	much, many
post	after
poster(o)	back, behind
presby(o)-	old age
proct(o)	anus, rectum
pseud(o)	false
psych(o)	mind
pulmon(o)	lung
pyel(o)	kidney
pyr(o)	fever
quadri	four
ren(o)	kidney
retro	behind, backward
rhin(o)	nose
-rrhage	bursting forth
salping(o)	fallopian tubes
sclero(o)	hard
-scope	instrument
-scopy	visual exam
somat(o)	body
sten(o)	narrow
supra-	above
tachy-	fast, rapid

continued

PREFIX–SUFFIX–ROOT	MEANING
therap(y)	treatment
therm(o)	heat
thorac(o)	chest
thromb(o)	blood clot
-tomy	incision
tox(o)	poison
trache(o)	trachea
-uria	urine
vas(o)	vessel
ven(o)	vein
vesic(o)	bladder

MEDICAL DICTIONARIES

In some programs, a good medical dictionary is a required text-book. If it is not a required text, it would be wise for you to invest in a good medical dictionary. There are many on the market, but find one that is comprehensive yet compact enough that you can easily carry it with you to the clinical area. If you can afford to buy a handheld personal digital assistant (PDA), buy the information in a "downloadable" format for it. The idea is to **have the dictionary with you when you are reading the patient's medical records and charts.**

When you are reading the patient's chart, do not skip over medical words you do not know. Look up the term as you read. The more you do this, the quicker you will begin to understand the language.

PRACTICE WITH MEDICAL TERMS

Break down the following terms to identify their meaning using the preceding table. See how many you can understand without even taking a medical terminology course! Although the translation is "literal," you can guess what the words mean. Check your answers in Appendix A.

1. anesthesia
2. dysphagia

3. malnutrition
4. tachycardia
5. antibacterial
6. dyspnea
7. quadriplegia
8. hyperplasia
9. hypodermic
10. dyspepsia
11. pericarditis
12. phlebotomy
13. oliguria
14. cystoscopy
15. laparoscopy
16. hystero salpingo-oopherectomy
17. angiography
18. otitis
19. tracheostomy
20. leukocytopenia

NOTES

NOTES

Math Review

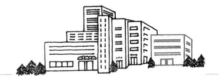

GETTING STARTED WITH MATH

You are probably asking yourself, "Why do I need math? I passed it in high school." Guess what, your second grade teacher was right when he or she said that you would need math for the rest of your life.

Math is a very important part of nursing. Nursing consists of many entities, and medication calculation is just one small part. Nurses do math every day at work. It could be a simple conversion or a difficult calculation in order to titrate a medication according to certain laboratory test results.

This chapter reviews the basic math skills you need. Each section of the chapter gives you building blocks to start the foundation for your math skills. It is important that you complete this chapter so you are prepared for your math exams in nursing school. It might seem like easy math problems to you, but you could miss a few because you do not remember how to figure out the problem. So, sit back, relax, and work your brain.

Keep your chin up. NO PAIN! NO GAIN!

MATH STUDY GUIDE

REDUCING FRACTIONS

Usually fractions are reduced to their lowest terms.

When reducing a fraction to its lowest terms, divide the numerator and denominator by the largest number that each is evenly divisible by.

Example 1: Reduce the following fraction: $\dfrac{8}{20}$

Solution: The numerator and denominator are evenly divisible by 4.

$$8 \div 4 = 2 \quad \text{and} \quad 20 \div 4 = 5$$

Therefore: $\dfrac{8}{20} = \dfrac{2}{5}$

Example 2: Reduce the following fraction: $\dfrac{65}{100}$

Solution: The numerator and denominator are evenly divisible by 5.

$$65 \div 5 = 13 \quad \text{and} \quad 100 \div 5 = 20$$

$$\dfrac{65}{100} = \dfrac{13}{20}$$

MULTIPLYING FRACTIONS

When multiplying fractions, multiply the numerators and then the denominators. If there is a mixed number be sure to change it into an improper fraction before multiplying. **_Reduce_** the fraction if necessary. You can reduce the fraction, if it is not in its lowest terms, before multiplying.

Example 1:

$$\frac{2}{3} \times \frac{5}{8}$$

Solution:

$$\frac{2 \times 5 = 10}{3 \times 8 = 24} = \frac{5}{12}$$

Example 2:

$$8 \times \frac{5}{8}$$

Solution:

$$8 \times \frac{5}{8} = \frac{40}{8} = 5$$

$$\frac{8}{1} \times \frac{5}{8} = \frac{40}{8} = 5$$

(Express whole numbers as a fraction by placing a one as the denominator.)

Example 3:

$$4\frac{1}{2} \times 2\frac{3}{4}$$

Solution:

$$4\frac{1}{2} = \frac{9}{2} \qquad 2\frac{3}{4} = \frac{11}{4}$$

$$\frac{9}{2} \times \frac{11}{4} = \frac{99}{8} = 12\frac{3}{8}$$

DIVIDING FRACTIONS

When dividing fractions, you need to invert the divisor (second fraction) and then multiply. Simplify prior to working out the problem. Reduce the fraction when necessary.

Example 1:

$$\frac{2}{3} \div \frac{6}{9}$$

Solution:

$$\frac{2 \times 9}{3 \times 6} = \frac{18}{24} = \frac{3}{4}$$

Example 2:

$$1\frac{2}{5} \div 2\frac{3}{5}$$

Solution:

$$1\frac{2}{5} = \frac{7}{5} \qquad 2\frac{3}{5} = \frac{13}{5}$$

$$\frac{7}{5} \times \frac{5}{13} = \frac{35}{65} = \frac{7}{13}$$

Example 3:

$$6 \div \frac{1}{3}$$

Solution:

$$\frac{6 \times 3}{1 \times 1} = \frac{18}{1} = 18$$

Example 4:

$\frac{1}{8}$ numerator
$\frac{1}{2}$ demoninator

Solution:

$$\frac{1}{8} \times \frac{2}{1} = \frac{2}{8} = \frac{1}{4}$$

MULTIPLYING DECIMALS

The main precaution when multiplying decimals is the placement of the decimal point in the answer.

Example 1:

$$0.25 \times 0.5 = 0.125$$

Solution:

$$\begin{array}{r} 0.25 \\ \times\ \ 0.5 \\ \hline 0.125 \end{array}$$

In this problem, the 0.25 has two numbers to the right of the decimal, and 0.5 has one number to the right; therefore, put the decimal point three places to the left in the product. Always put a zero to the left of the decimal to emphasize the decimal when the answer is less than one.

Example 2:

$$1.8 \times 0.35 = 0.63$$

Solution:

$$\begin{array}{r} 1.80 \\ \times\ 0.35 \\ \hline 0.63 \end{array}$$

Start the problem by lining up the numbers on the right. Do not pay attention to the decimals until the end of the problem. Multiply the numbers as if they were whole numbers. Count how many numbers there are to the right of the decimal. This is where you will put your decimal in the final answer. Always put the decimal point in the answer to the left by using the **total** number of decimal places after the decimal point in the problem. Add as many zeros as you need to correctly place the decimal.

$$\begin{array}{r} 0.35 \\ \times\ 0.21 \\ \hline 735 \end{array} \quad \text{answer} = 0.0735$$

In this problem, there are four numbers after all the decimal points. Therefore, put the decimal point four places to the left in the product. Add one zero to allow correct placement of the decimal point.

DIVIDING DECIMALS

To divide decimals, simplify the fraction before doing the actual division. The first step will do away with the decimal point completely. When removing the decimal from the fraction, move the decimal the same number of spaces to the right in the numerator and the denominator. A zero can be added to accomplish this.

Example 1:

$\dfrac{0.35}{0.125}$ becomes $\dfrac{350}{125}$

Example 2:

$\dfrac{2.5}{3}$ becomes $\dfrac{25}{30}$

Example 3:

$\dfrac{.60}{.15}$ becomes $\dfrac{60}{15}$

Example 4:

$\dfrac{5.5}{0.63}$ becomes $\dfrac{550}{63}$

Reducing fractions that end in zeros

When both the numerator and denominator end in zero(s), you can reduce the fraction by crossing off the same amount of zeros in each number.

Example 1:

$$\frac{2400}{100} = \frac{24}{1}$$

Example 2:

$$\frac{600}{250} = \frac{60}{25}$$

Example 3:

$$\frac{65000}{25000} = \frac{65}{25}$$

Example 4:

$$\frac{3000}{1400} = \frac{30}{14}$$

Rounding off to the nearest tenth

When rounding to the nearest tenth, carry the division to the hundredths place. If the number in the hundredths place is 5 or greater, increase the number in the tenths place by one.

Examples:

$0.88 = 0.9$ $1.63 = 1.6$

$0.63 = 0.6$ $0.18 = 0.2$

When rounding to the **nearest hundredth, carry** the division to the thousandth. Again, if the number in the thousandths place is 5 or greater, the number in the hundredths place is increased by one.

Examples:

$0.632 = 0.63$ $0.622 = 0.62$

$0.888 = 0.89$ $1.666 = 1.67$

In the first example, the number in the *thousandths column* is 2; therefore, the number in the hundredths column stays the same.

$0.624 = 0.62$

ADDING FRACTIONS

In order to add fractions, the denominators need to be the same. If the denominators are not the same, you must change the fraction(s) utilizing the least common denominator.

Example 1:

$$\frac{1}{8} + \frac{1}{3} =$$

Solution:

$$\frac{1}{8} = \frac{3}{24} \quad \text{and} \quad \frac{1}{3} = \frac{8}{24}$$

$$\frac{3}{24} + \frac{8}{24} = \frac{11}{24}$$

Example 2:

$$\frac{1}{6} + \frac{1}{8} + \frac{11}{3} =$$

Solution:

$$\frac{4}{24} + \frac{3}{24} + \frac{88}{24} = \frac{95}{24} = 3\frac{23}{24}$$

CHANGING FRACTIONS AND DECIMALS TO PERCENTAGES

In order to change a fraction into a percentage you must *multiply* the fraction by 100, reduce, and add the percent sign.

Example 1:

$$\frac{2}{3} =$$

$$\frac{2}{3} \times \frac{100}{1} = \frac{200}{3} = 67\%$$

Example 2:

$$6\frac{3}{4} =$$

$$6\frac{3}{4} = \frac{27}{4} \times \frac{100}{1} = \frac{2700}{4} = 675\%$$

When **changing a decimal** into a **percentage,** move the decimal point two places to the right. You can add zeros if necessary. Remember to place the percent sign at the end.

$$0.62 = 62\%$$

$$8.6 = 860\%$$

$$0.525 = 52\frac{1}{2}\% = 52.5\%$$

You may also change the decimal into a fraction, and then follow the steps to change the fraction into a percentage. If the remainder is not a whole number, then express the answer in a fraction, to the nearest whole percent or the nearest tenth of a percent.

To **change a percentage back to a decimal,** drop the percent sign, and move the decimal **two** spaces to the left.

$$50\% = 0.50$$

$$2.8\% = 0.028$$

Converting percentages to fractions

A percentage is the portion of 100 considered in the problem. The term *percent* refers to the hundredths column. A percentage, converted into a fraction, will always contain 100 as the denominator.

$$6\% = \frac{6}{100}$$

A whole number (80%), fraction $\left(\frac{1}{2}\%\right)$, mixed number $\left(2\frac{1}{2}\%\right)$, and decimal (.5%) may be expressed as a percentage. Therefore, a percentage can be expressed in different forms without changing the value.

$$10\% = \frac{10}{100} = \frac{1}{10}$$

$$\frac{1}{3}\% = \frac{1}{3} \div \frac{100}{1} = \frac{1}{3} \times \frac{1}{100} = \frac{1}{300}$$

 Take a Slow, Deep Breath.

PRACTICE PROBLEMS

Reduce the following fractions into lowest terms. Check your answers in Appendix B.

1. $\dfrac{20}{30}$ _____

2. $\dfrac{8}{64}$ _____

3. $\dfrac{50}{130}$ ____

4. $\dfrac{120}{160}$ ____

5. $\dfrac{16}{24}$ ____

6. $\dfrac{14}{196}$ ____

7. $\dfrac{10}{16}$ ____

8. $\dfrac{48}{72}$ ____

9. $\dfrac{20}{60}$ ____

10. $\dfrac{6}{36}$ ____

Multiply the following fractions.

11. $\dfrac{1}{4} \times \dfrac{2}{25} =$

12. $\dfrac{2}{3} \times \dfrac{1}{4} =$

13. $6 \times 3\dfrac{3}{4} =$

14. $\dfrac{1}{2} \times \dfrac{3}{4} =$

15. $8 \times \dfrac{11}{2} =$

16. $\dfrac{8}{6} \times \dfrac{32}{4} =$

17. $\dfrac{10}{15} \times \dfrac{3}{2} =$

18. $\dfrac{11}{3} \times \dfrac{6}{9} =$

19. $2\dfrac{2}{3} \times \dfrac{1}{4} =$

20. $10 \times \dfrac{3}{5} =$

Divide the following fractions.

21. $\dfrac{22}{3} \div 4\dfrac{1}{3} =$

22. $\dfrac{1}{2} \div \dfrac{3}{4} =$

23. $\dfrac{2}{3} \div \dfrac{4}{5} =$

27. $\dfrac{10}{25} \div \dfrac{10}{5} =$

24. $2 \div \dfrac{1}{18} =$

28. $4\dfrac{1}{2} \div \dfrac{7}{10} =$

25. $3 \div \dfrac{2}{10} =$

29. $6\dfrac{2}{3} \div \dfrac{1}{18} =$

26. $\dfrac{4}{3} \div \dfrac{3}{6} =$

30. $\dfrac{6}{3} \div \dfrac{6}{3} =$

Multiply the following problems.

31. $0.55 \times 0.3 =$

32. $2.3 \times 0.16 =$

33. $4.8 \times 2.1 =$

34. $3.5 \times 6.2 =$

35. $1.2 \times 0.02 =$

36. $6.35 \times 2.3 =$

37. $0.6 \times 0.08 =$

38. $11.6 \times 1.2 =$

39. $2 \times 0.05 =$

40. $0.2 \times 0.18 =$

Eliminate the decimal.

41. $\dfrac{0.5}{0.05} =$

46. $\dfrac{0.1}{.04} =$

42. $\dfrac{1.5}{0.3} =$

47. $\dfrac{0.5}{0.12} =$

43. $\dfrac{12.75}{4.5} =$

48. $\dfrac{0.8}{24} =$

44. $\dfrac{6.3}{0.6} =$

49. $\dfrac{20}{0.2} =$

45. $\dfrac{3.75}{0.5} =$

50. $\dfrac{7.45}{0.3} =$

Divide to the nearest tenth.

51. $\dfrac{2.5}{1.2} =$

53. $\dfrac{6}{1.2} =$

52. $\dfrac{0.8}{0.4} =$

54. $\dfrac{2.8}{1.2} =$

55. $\dfrac{0.5}{2.2} =$

57. $\dfrac{0.12}{.125} =$

56. $\dfrac{0.7}{0.22} =$

58. $\dfrac{2.6}{2.8} =$

Divide the fractions, and round the answer to the nearest hundredth.

59. $\dfrac{16}{1.5} =$

69. $\dfrac{0.64}{0.8} =$

60. $\dfrac{160,000}{200,000} =$

70. $\dfrac{650}{10,000} =$

61. $\dfrac{10}{12.5} =$

71. $\dfrac{0.05}{0.15} =$

62. $\dfrac{70}{280} =$

72. $\dfrac{0.5}{1.25} =$

63. $\dfrac{22}{0.2} =$

73. $\dfrac{75}{150} =$

64. $\dfrac{0.1}{1.2} =$

74. $\dfrac{1650}{1500} =$

65. $\dfrac{0.20}{0.3} =$

75. $\dfrac{0.135}{0.5} =$

66. $\dfrac{2.2}{6.2} =$

76. $\dfrac{800}{1600} =$

67. $\dfrac{0.125}{0.4} =$

77. $\dfrac{5.5}{24.2} =$

68. $\dfrac{0.12}{0.24} =$

78. $\dfrac{2.02}{6.2} =$

Add the following fractions.

79. $\dfrac{1}{4} + \dfrac{3}{6} + \dfrac{2}{3} =$

80. $\dfrac{2}{3} + \dfrac{5}{8} + 2\dfrac{1}{3} =$

81. $\dfrac{1}{2} + \dfrac{2}{3} =$

82. $\dfrac{1}{5} + \dfrac{1}{4} =$

83. $\dfrac{3}{4} + \dfrac{1}{2} + 2\dfrac{2}{3} =$

84. $1\dfrac{1}{13} + \dfrac{2}{2} + \dfrac{1}{2} =$

85. $2\dfrac{1}{8} + \dfrac{1}{2} =$

86. $\dfrac{2}{3} + \dfrac{1}{2} =$

87. $\dfrac{1}{18} + \dfrac{1}{6} =$

88. $\dfrac{6}{10} + \dfrac{1}{5} + \dfrac{1}{2} =$

Take Another Breath. You Are Almost Done!

Change the fractions to percentages.

89. $\dfrac{3}{5}$ _____

90. $2\dfrac{2}{3}$ _____

91. $\dfrac{1}{3}$ _____

92. $\dfrac{2}{3}$ _____

93. $\dfrac{1}{2}$ _____

Change the decimal to a percentage.

94. .63 _____

95. 1.25 _____

96. 0.08 _____

97. 6.25 _____

98. 0.005 _____

Change the percentages to decimals.

99. 20% _____

100. 65% _____

101. 550% _____

102. 100% _____

103. 6% _____

Express the following percentages in reduced fractions.

104. 50% _____

105. 70% _____

106. 1% _____

107. 5% _____

108. 24% _____

Conversions

Volume

1 tsp	=	5 ml
1 TBSP	=	15 ml
1 ounce	=	30 ml

1 cup	=	240 ml
1 pint	=	946 ml
1 liter	=	1000 ml

Weight

1 mg	=	1000 mcg
1 g	=	1000 mg
1 grain	=	60 mg
1 kg	=	2.2 lbs
1 liter of water	=	1 kg
1 oz	=	28 g
1 kilogram	=	1000 g

$lbs = kg \times 2.2$ $\qquad$ $kg = lbs \times 0.45$

$°F = (°C \times 1.8) + 32$ $\qquad$ $°C = (°F - 32) \times \dfrac{5}{9}$

$inches = cm \times 0.394$ $\qquad$ $cm = inches \times 2.54$

Common IV Rates

Volume in Bag	Time to Infuse	Rate
250 ml	2 hours	125 ml
100 ml	60 mins	100 ml
100 ml	30 mins	200 ml
50 ml	30 mins	100 ml

 STAYING FOCUSED

In order to have an optimal study session, you need to stay focused on your studying. If you find your mind wandering, try these hints to help you focus:

1. Make your study area brighter.
2. Take breaks when you need to.
3. Make sure your study area is comfortable.
4. Let family and friends know not to bother you during your study time.

NOTES

NOTES

Test Taking Techniques

AFTER BUILDING BRICK #8, THE STUDENT WILL BE ABLE TO:

- Define the steps needed in test preparation.
- Develop skills needed for taking multiple-choice tests.

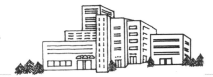

PREPARING FOR A TEST

THROUGHOUT THE TERM:

1. Take notes, highlight, and review all assigned readings.

2. Review and edit your notes from lectures and assigned readings within 24 hours of the lecture.

3. Write and answer study questions from each unit on a weekly basis.

4. Organize your notes, handouts, and study questions regularly. Use an accordion-style folder to keep papers organized neatly.

A WEEK OR TWO WEEKS BEFORE THE TEST:

1. Outline the main topics.
2. Use good time management skills to plan your study time.
3. Do not study the information all at once.
4. Spread the information into sections and span it over a few days.
5. Meet with your study group at least three times before the test.
6. Make up test questions and study flash cards to prepare for objective questions.
7. Write out answers to essay questions that you think could be asked.

"I Can Do This and I Will!"

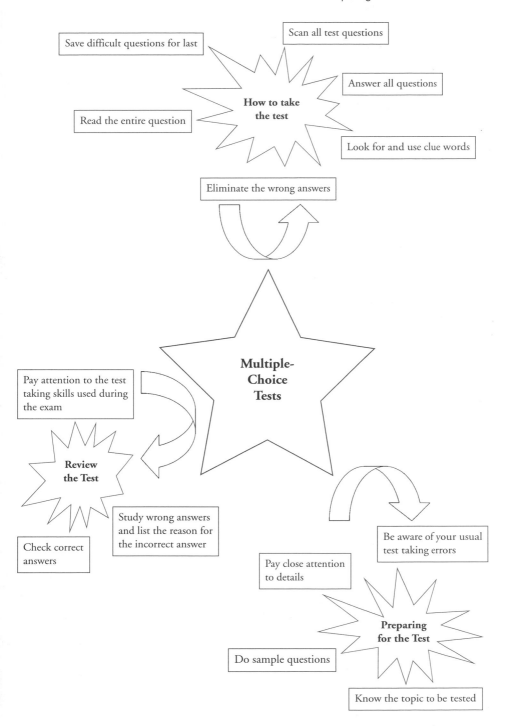

Save difficult questions for last

Scan all test questions

How to take the test

Answer all questions

Read the entire question

Look for and use clue words

Eliminate the wrong answers

Multiple-Choice Tests

Pay attention to the test taking skills used during the exam

Review the Test

Study wrong answers and list the reason for the incorrect answer

Check correct answers

Be aware of your usual test taking errors

Pay close attention to details

Preparing for the Test

Do sample questions

Know the topic to be tested

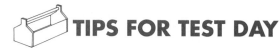

TIPS FOR TEST DAY

- Rest. Get at least six hours of sleep the night before the test.
- Eat a small meal before the test.
- Avoid caffeinated drinks and foods that will over stimulate you.
- Exercise. It can invigorate your mind by increasing cerebral function.
- Have pencils, erasers, calculator, and any other materials needed for the test.
- Get to class on time without rushing.
- Read test directions carefully. Listen to verbal instruction.
- Budget your time efficiently.
- Skim through the test for levels of difficult questions.
- Flag questions you are not sure of the answer.

When finished:
- Reread instructions to be sure you followed them correctly.
- Be sure you have answered all the questions.
- Check questions flagged for further review.
- Review all questions.

Good Luck!

MEMORY STEPS

1. Acronyms: Words created from the initial letters of the series of words.
   Example: There are four blood types: A, B, O, and AB.
      Any
      Other
      Bloods
      Abnormal

2. Acoustics: A sentence made by using the first letters of the key words in a list of items to create words or a sentence that helps trigger your memory. Example: The three initial signs of diabetes are:

Polydipsia	Papa's
Polyphagia	Pizza
Polyuria	Pie

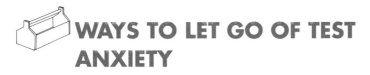

WAYS TO LET GO OF TEST ANXIETY

If you freeze during tests and get questions wrong when you know the right answers, you may have test taking anxiety. Try the following simple techniques:

1. Mentally yell "STOP!"—it will focus you back to the present.
2. Visualize success.
3. Praise yourself, "I am relaxed, I am doing a great job."
4. Take a few slow, deep breaths.
5. Sit comfortably and close your eyes for a few minutes and relax your muscles.
6. If these techniques don't help, talk to your school counselor for further suggestions.

PARTS TO MULTIPLE-CHOICE QUESTIONS

Item = entire multiple-choice question

Stem = statement that asks the question

Options = possible responses offered by the item

Correct answer = option that answers the question being asked

Distracter = incorrect answer(s)

Example:

1. What should a nurse do immediately before performing any procedure?
   a. Shut the door   DISTRACTER
   a. Wash his or her hands   CORRECT ANSWER

     a. Close the curtain   DISTRACTER

     a. Drape the patient   DISTRACTER

2. When providing care to a patient with a nasogastric tube, the nurse recognizes that the tube is in the:

     c. stomach.   CORRECT ANSWER

     d. bronchi.   DISTRACTER

     e. trachea.   DISTRACTER

     f. duodenum.   DISTRACTER

TYPES OF STEMS

Complete sentence: The stem poses a question and ends with a question mark.

Example:

What should be the first action of a nurse when a fire alarm rings in a health care facility?

    a. Close all the doors on the unit.

    b. Take an extinguisher to the fire scene.

    c. Move clients laterally toward the stairs.

    d. Determine if it is a fire drill or a real fire.

Correct answer: **A.** Rationale: A closed door provides for client safety.

Incomplete sentence: The stem forms the beginning portion of a sentence. The sentence becomes complete when combined with the correct option in the item.

Example: To *better* understand what a client is saying, the nurse should:

    a. demonstrate interest.

    b. listen carefully.

    c. remain silent.

    d. employ touch.

Correct answer: **B.** Rationale: Attentive listening is important so the nurse can pick up key words and identify emotional themes within the message.

Positive polarity: The stem is concerned with the truth. The correct answer accurately relates to the statement.

Example:

Which intervention most accurately supports the concept of informed consent?

    a.   Obtaining the client's signature.

    b.   Explaining what is being done and why.

    c.   Involving the family in the teaching plan.

    d.   Teaching preoperative deep breathing and coughing.

Correct answer: **B.** Rationale: The client's knowledge and understanding of what is to be done, why it is to be done, and what the outcomes will be constitute informed consent.

Negative polarity: The stem is concerned with what is false and usually contains words such as "except," "not," "contraindicated," or "least." Look for exceptions, detect errors, or identify interventions that are unacceptable or contraindicated.

Example:

On what part of the body should the nurse avoid using soap when bathing a client?

    a.   Eyes

    b.   Back

    c.   Under breasts

    d.   Abdomen

Correct answer: **A.** Rationale. Soaps usually contain sodium or potassium salts of fatty acids, which are irritating and can injure the eyes.

TYPES OF OPTIONS

Sentence options: Stem + option = sentence. Option completes the sentence begun in the stem.

Example:

The primary etiology of obesity is a:

    a.   lack of balance in the variety of nutrients.

    b.   glandular disorder that prevents weight loss.

    c.   caloric intake that exceeds metabolic needs.

    d.   psychological problem that causes overeating.

Correct answer: **C.** Rationale: If the body ingests more calories than it requires for energy, the calories convert to adipose tissue, which causes weight gain.

Incomplete sentence option: Usually a phrase or a group of related words, this option conveys an idea or concept though not in a complete sentence.

Example:

When should mouth care be administered to an unconscious client?

    a.   Whenever necessary

    b.   Every 4 hours

    c.   Once a shift

    d.   Twice a day

Correct answer: **A.** Rationale: Unconscious clients usually have dry mucous membranes of the oral cavity because they frequently breathe through the mouth, and are not drinking fluids. Oral hygiene is required whenever necessary.

Word options: A single word, a noun, pronoun, verb, or adjective that conveys information, can also be an option.

Example:

Which word best describes feelings associated with a child in Erikson's stage of autonomy versus shame and doubt?

    a.   Hers

    b.   Mine

    c.   Theirs

    d.   Nobody's

Correct answer: **B.** Rationale: Toddlers are developing a sense of autonomy and are discovering the difference between independence and dependence. They are concerned about themselves and their mastery over their environment.

BECOMING A WISE TEST TAKER

Tests or examinations in the health professions can be very anxiety provoking until you become wise to how the instructors ask questions. The information you are learning in the classroom and reading in textbooks is only as important as your ability to **apply** the information to patient care situations. Remember, when you take notes during a lecture, the test will not usually ask you to list back the information in the same manner as it was presented. For example, if the instructor tells you about a medication that affects blood clotting (anticoagulant), you, most likely, will not be asked to merely list the drug. You are more likely to receive a patient care situation where you must answer what actions a nurse must take because the patient is receiving an anticoagulant.

Nursing is a **practice** discipline. This means you must be able to apply the theory taught in class to patient care or nursing practice situations. We all know people who are "book smart" but cannot apply what they learn to situations. You must know the theory and be able to use it to provide patient care.

Your instructors write application questions in order to prepare you for the even bigger test down the road following graduation—the certification test for licensure. To be licensed as a registered nurse, you must be able to pass the National Council Licensure Examination for Registered Nurses (NCLEX-RN).

Most schools require instructors to write **behavioral objectives** for their lesson plans to teach the content in a course. A behavioral objective specifies what a learner will be able to do after a teaching session. Objectives also help to guide the student by providing information about what the student will be able to do as a result of the class. Examinations should be based on the objectives for the class or teaching session. For example, an instructor writes the following objective:

The student will describe the care for a patient with sickle cell disease.

Therefore, an exam will expect the learner to show that he or she knows what the care of a patient with sickle cell disease entails. A sample question related to this objective could be:

Cindy Smith comes to the emergency department in sickle cell crisis. Which of the following interventions should the nurse consider a priority?

a. Draw blood for a blood count

b. Administer oxygen

c. Provide for genetic counseling

d. Administer red blood cells

Correct answer: **B.** Rationale: Oxygen is one of the primary needs of a patient in sickle cell crisis. The other choices are important interventions but not a priority for the patient first seen in the emergency department. Notice, the question does not merely ask the learner to list the care for a patient with sickle cell disease; rather, the learner is asked what the priority is. In this example, the learner must know what the care is, and what is most important in an acute care situation.

▪ *TEST TIP:* Review the unit objectives. They provide guidance on what to study for exams.

If the instructor permits you to write in the test booklet, it is wise to underline the important parts of the question. Many times the question includes a situation. You need to be able to identify the important information provided in the question.

Cindy Smith comes to the *emergency department* in *sickle cell crisis.* Which of the following *interventions* should the nurse consider a *priority*?

a. Draw blood for a blood count

b. Administer oxygen

c. Provide for genetic counseling

d. Administer red blood cells

In the preceding question, it is important to know exactly what is being asked. By underlining "emergency department," "sickle cell crisis," "interventions," and "priority," you should have all the clues to help answer the question. It asks what the priority (most important) intervention is in the emergency (acute) phase of sickle cell disease (crisis). Underlining the important aspects of the question helps you to focus on the answer. Before you even look at the choices, try to figure out the answer, and then quickly look for it in the choices.

■ *TEST TIP:* Underline the important aspects of the question to determine exactly what is being asked.

Become aware of key words or phrases used in questions. Instructors often use words such as "**best**," "**most important**," "**priority**," and "**first**" to determine if you know how to distinguish among a list of things you would do to care for a patient. Notice that these types of questions are not just asking what you would do in a particular situation but in what order you would do it. In the preceding question, it is appropriate to provide all the interventions listed for a client in sickle cell crisis. The question, however, asks what you should do first in an emergency situation.

■ *TEST TIP:* Look for key words that indicate all interventions are correct, but that one is best or should be done first.

"Reading into the question" is one of the problems that most beginning students have with application or nursing care questions. This occurs when the student thinks about too many facts that really are not included in the question. When answering questions, **only consider the information provided.** Do not think about facts outside of the question. The previous underlining technique discussed could help to keep you focused.

Example:

Nurse Joan is caring for Mr. Smith, who had a stroke two days ago. He has a sudden onset of breathing difficulties. His vital signs are 140/70, 88, 28. What action should Nurse Joan take first?

a. Recheck the vital signs

b. Request an EKG

c. Elevate the head of the bed

d. Notify the physician

Correct answer: **C.** Rationale: There is no need to recheck the vital signs at this time. Eventually, an EKG could be needed. Quickly elevating the head of the bed could relieve the breathing difficulties. Maintaining an airway, breathing, and circulation (the ABCs) are always a priority. Notification of the physician is important, but elevating the head of the bed could help with the dyspnea. **Do not start to add facts or questions like whether he has chest pain, pain in his left arm, etc. Only deal with the facts**

contained in the question. His respiratory rate is elevated and he has difficulty breathing!

▪ *TEST TIP:* Do not "read into the question" facts that are not included in the situation.

When taking exams, it is important to pay attention to negatively phrased questions. Words like "least likely," "except," "least helpful," or "avoid" are all examples of negative words used in questions. When you see these words, make sure you underline them to remind you that the question is focusing on a negative response. An example of this type of question follows:

A patient has hypertension. Which of the following foods should the patient be taught to avoid?

   a.   Carrots

   b.   Bananas

   c.   Canned soup

   d.   Raisins

Correct answer: **C.** Rationale: Canned soups are high in sodium, which can cause fluid retention and an increase in blood pressure. The other foods do not have the same effect. Notice that the word "avoid" prompts you to choose the food that is "bad" for the patient.

▪ *TEST TIP:* Pay attention to negatively written questions. Look for key words such as "avoid," "except," "least likely," etc.

ANALYZING YOUR EXAM PERFORMANCE

If you are not performing as well as you think you should on exams, you need to analyze what the problem is.

• Are you really spending quality time studying? Are you easily distracted? Do you need to change the environment in which you are studying? Some students say, "I don't know how I did so poorly on the exam. I studied all night." When they analyze how they are studying, they find they spent half of the time with interruptions.

• Do you have many other responsibilities competing for your time such as family or work? Perhaps, you will need to cut back on work. Perhaps, you need to have a heart-to-heart talk with family members to enlist their support particularly when you have an upcoming exam.

• How well are you taking notes? If you are not sure, compare them with others in the class. Show them to an instructor for an opinion on how thorough you are taking notes and getting the information. Consider tape-recording the lectures. Make sure you ask permission of the instructor first.

• Are you using the objectives on the syllabus or outline to focus your study sessions?

• Do you review your notes on a daily basis instead of waiting to the last minute to study and then cram the night before?

• Do you have an abnormal anxiety with regard to exams? If so, you need to start taking steps to curb the anxiety. Perhaps relaxation techniques can help. If the anxiety is extreme, you may need to seek out a counselor.

By doing some introspection and answering these questions, perhaps you can find the root of the problem. You need to tackle this early in the program or you will find yourself floundering every time you are in an exam situation. Fix the problems early in the program so that your anxiety about exams will diminish and you will bolster your confidence.

TEST ANALYSIS TOOL (TAT)

Okay, you got your first test back. How did you do? Review each question thoroughly and ask yourself: "What were my difficulties in choosing the correct answers?" Reflect on this and answer the following questions as accurately as you can to help analyze your test performance.

1. Did I feel confident and prepared while taking the test?

   Yes   No

2. Did I finish the test with enough time for review.

   Yes   No

3. Did I feel calm and in control while taking the test?

   Yes   No

4. Did I change any of my answers? If so, did I answer the question right?

   Yes   No

5. Did I understand every question?

   Yes   No

If you answered "Yes" to the preceding questions: Good Work!!! You are using the proper tools for successful test taking. If you answered "No" to any of the questions, follow these blueprints:

- Get a good night's sleep.
- Arrive to class early so you can relax before test time.
- Wear comfortable clothing.
- Read all directions carefully before beginning the test.
- Skim through the test and estimate how long each section will take.
- Watch the clock.
- Answer the questions you are sure of first and come back to the more difficult ones later.
- Be careful to mark your answer sheet carefully.
- Read all of the choices before choosing your final answer.
- If you change your answer, base it on solid facts.
- If you're just not sure of the answer, make an educated guess.
- Do not cram the night before.
- Review Chapter 4, "Study Skills."
- Review Chapter 8, "Test Taking Techniques."
- Focus, stay in control.
- Concentrate only on the test.
- Avoid minor distractions by sitting away from a door or window.
- Double-check your test for any careless errors before turning it in.

TEST TRACKING TOOL

Name_____ Class_____ Goal Grade_____

EXAM	POINTS EARNED	TOTAL POINTS OFFERED	AREAS TO IMPROVE

This tool will help you monitor your progress toward your goal grade and focus on the areas you need to improve.

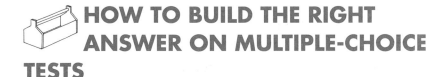

HOW TO BUILD THE RIGHT ANSWER ON MULTIPLE-CHOICE TESTS

1. Find key words and underline them.
2. Use your first "gut feeling."
3. Most answers that contain "probably," "sometimes," and "some" are usually right.
4. The most complicated answer is almost always correct.
5. Mark your answers on the answer sheet when doing the question.
6. If using a Scantron, make sure your mark corresponds to the question you are answering.
7. Do not read too much into the question.
8. Answers that are similar tend to both be wrong.

9. Look for wrong answers when you do not know the right one.

10. Read every answer.

11. Recheck your answers.

A WORD ABOUT TEST REVIEWS . . .

• If offered a test review, take advantage of it! Attending a test review helps you to understand the correct answers. You are anxious to find out your grade, but do not stop there!

• It is just as important to understand why the wrong answers are wrong, as it is to know what the right answer was.

• Try to understand the concept being tested. You will probably see the concept tested again in another way . . . perhaps even on the final exam!

• If you disagree with the answer and think that another choice on an exam could be correct, do your homework. Do not argue with the instructor in front of other students. Approach the instructor after class or make an appointment to discuss the question. Take "evidence" to the instructor that supports your answer by showing him or her text page numbers.

• If you really have not grasped the material, make an appointment to see the instructor to discuss the material. Make the appointment as soon as possible after the exam.

• If you perform poorly on an exam, do not wait until the end of the semester to ask for help. It could be too late for remediation and could lead to course failure. Instructors want to see that you are interested and are making an effort to understand the material. Most instructors will do everything they can to help you IF you demonstrate effort on your part.

NOTES

NOTES

Now you are ready to begin constructing your future for success in nursing school. You have learned the basic building bricks that you will need to be successful. We hope that you enjoyed the book and wish you the best of luck in your marvelous and exciting future.

Good Luck!

Dona, Christy, and Carol

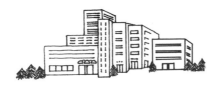

Appendix A

Answers to Practice with Medical Terms

1.	anesthesia	absence of feeling or sensation
2.	dysphagia	difficulty with eating
3.	malnutrition	poor nutrition
4.	tachycardia	rapid heart rate
5.	antibacterial	against bacteria
6.	dyspnea	difficulty breathing
7.	quadriplegia	"four" paralysis (paralysis of four limbs)
8.	hyperplasia	excessive growth
9.	hypodermic	below the skin
10.	dyspepsia	difficulty with digestion
11.	pericarditis	inflammation around the heart
12.	phlebotomy	incision into the vein; usually to draw blood
13.	oliguria	scanty urine
14.	cystoscopy	visual exam of the bladder
15.	laparoscopy	visual exam of the abdomen
16.	hystero salpingo-oopherectomy	removal of the uterus, fallopian tubes, and ovary
17.	angiography	a record or test of a blood vessel
18.	otitis	inflammation of the ear
19.	tracheostomy	opening into the trachea
20.	leukocytopenia	deficiency of white blood cells

Appendix B

Answers to the Practice Problems

1. 2/3
2. 1/8
3. 5/13
4. ¾
5. 2/3
6. 1/14
7. 5/8
8. 2/3
9. 1/3
10. 1/6
11. 1/50
12. 1/6
13. 22½
14. 3/8
15. 44
16. 10 2/3
17. 1
18. 8/9
19. 2/3
20. 6
21. 8/13
22. 2/3
23. 5/6
24. 36
25. 15
26. 2 2/3
27. 1/5
28. 6 3/7

29. 120
30. 1
31. 0.165
32. 0.368
33. 10.08
34. 21.7
35. 0.024
36. 14.605
37. 0.048
38. 13.92
39. 0.1
40. 0.036
41. 50/5 or 10
42. 15/30
43. 1275/450
44. 63/6
45. 375/50
46. 10/4
47. 50/12
48. 80/24
49. 20/20
50. 745/30
51. 2.1
52. 2
53. 5
54. 2.3
55. 0.2
56. 3.2

57. 1.0
58. 0.9
59. 10.67
60. 0.8
61. 0.8
62. 0.25
63. 110
64. 0.08
65. 0.67
66. 0.35
67. 0.31
68. 0.5
69. 0.8
70. 0.07
71. 0.33
72. 0.4
73. 0.5
74. 1.1
75. 0.27
76. 0.5
77. 0.23
78. 0.33
79. 28/24
80. 87/24
81. 7/6
82. 9/20
83. 47 1/12
84. 2 15/26

85. 21/8	93. 50%	101. 5.50
86. 7/6	94. 63%	102. 1.0
87. 2/9	95. 125%	103. 0.06
88. 3/10	96. 8%	104. ½
89. 60%	97. 625%	105. 7/10
90. 2.67	98. 0.5%	106. 1/10
91. 33.3%	99. 0.20	107. 1/20
92. 66.7% or 67%	100. 0.65	108. 6/25

Index